Contents

Introduction

Shingles disease, caused by the varicella zoster virus, is a debilitating, acute illness that affects at least 50% of individuals 60 years of age or older. While the varicella zoster virus has been present in human history for centuries, scientists and doctors often confused it with other types of rash-creating diseases such as small pox and leprosy. Caused by the same relatively common virus that causes chicken pox; shingles presents physically with a series of painful, swollen blisters usually on one side of the body. In addition, shingles affects the individual neurologically. Because of this dual mechanism of presentation, shingles can be both intensely painful and embarrassing.

Historically, chicken pox was long viewed as a reasonably benign childhood disease that left, at most, some scars in its wake. After the chicken pox ebb, varicella zoster virus remains, lurking deep within the nerve cells in the body. While they lay dormant, the virus can reactivate quickly, resulting in a shingles outbreak. Shingles is a more painful disease that can sometimes result in sustained, painful sensations. The longer the lifespan of humans, the greater the chance that their varicella zoster virus infection will slip out of its dormancy and into disease.

While older adults contract shingles at a much higher rate than do their young adult or adolescent counterparts, shingles can occur at any point in life. Shingles can affect people at all stages in their lives, and it can develop at any point after exposure to the varicella virus. With the advent of varicella vaccination, some controversy has erupted about the virus, the vaccine and its link to shingles outbreaks. Education about varicella zoster virus can be helpful in quick identification and treatment that may mitigate the symptoms of this inconvenient and painful disease.

Varicella Zoster Virus

Varicella zoster virus (VZV) causes shingles. VZV belongs to the same viral family as herpes simplex, but the two present and are transmitted in completely different manners. People who have shingles should be reassured that their infection is not like herpes at all. VZV is a double-stranded DNA virus, which means that upon introduction to the human body, the virus must journey into the host's cell nuclei in order to begin manufacturing of more viruses. The cell that the virus chooses is extremely specific because it must match its viral body with receptors on the cell surface. VZV can infect many different body cells and as it reproduces, it exponentially increases in amount. Eventually VZV ends up in the nervous tissue, where the immune system cells are not permitted to go.

Because it is a double-stranded DNA virus, VZV is relatively stable. As it replicates, it can undergo division easily and without much chance of mutation. This is extremely helpful for doctors and scientists as they struggle to prevent the disease through vaccination and medication because an ever-shifting virus is extremely difficult to treat. VZV has not changed much at all in the time that scientists have been studying it. As a result, the treatments that were effective when doctors began using chemotherapeutic agents are the same medications that are currently being used to treat the virus.

VZV becomes introduced into the body through the respiratory tract. Usually, this is through airborne particles being inhaled into the lunch or coming in close physical contact with the virus. The body

4

absorbs VZV through the lining of the trachea or the bronchioles and then immediately migrates through the lymphatic system to the skin cells. This process takes about 14 days and is called the incubation period. After the incubation period, VZV targets the skin cells. The first time one is exposed to it, varicella expresses itself in the childhood disease chicken pox.

VZV is a crafty virus—it uses the cell's machinery and energy to create its copies. Essentially, it robs the cell of its ability to function in any manner except to create more viruses. VZV uses the cell's enzymes, energy source (ATP) and messenger RNA and other components to invade the body. Upon introduction to the cell's nuclei, VZV begins an assembly line type replication in which it uses the host's DNA polymerase, an enzyme that creates DNA, to create thousands of identical copies of itself. Once the nucleus is heavy with replicated copies of the VZV, the cell breaks apart and causes the viruses to be released into the surrounding tissues, eventually making its way into the bloodstream where the virus can travel throughout the body.

After the primary infection of chicken pox resolves (usually about two weeks) the virus migrates yet again to the body's nerve cells. Specifically, it moves into the nuclei of the nerve cells in the trigeminal nerve or the dorsal root ganglia. In these nerves, it lay dormant, waiting to become active again in the body. The dorsal root ganglia are sensory neurons, meaning that they connect to one or more dermatomes or skin areas of the body and are responsible for the sensations that are felt on or in the skin. The trigeminal nerve is responsible for enervating the eye.

Upon reactivation, which can occur for a variety of reasons discussed later, VZV begins to migrate through the neural connection to the dermatome associated with the particular nerve in which the virus has lain dormant. At the site of the skin cells, VZV creates clusters of painful blisters referred to as shingles. If the reactivated virus is in the trigeminal nerve, then it is most likely to reactivate in the ophthalmic areas of the nerve and lead to ocular zoster, which is shingles in the eye region.

The Immune System's Response

When varicella zoster virus invades the body, circulating cells in the blood stream, lymphatic system and mucous cells identify the virus as an organism that does not belong in the body. Cells that are specially designed to identify the invaders go to work the instant they come into a non-self cell or organism. Immediately upon recognizing that the VZV has invaded the body, special kinds of white blood cells called lymphocytes are ready to fight the organism.

Lymphocytes come in two varieties: B-cells and T-cells. All lymphocytes begin their lives in the bone marrow, where they are differentiated from other leukocytes. The B-cells become mature in the bone marrow (which is why they are called "B" cells), and the T-cells move on to the thymus to become mature (which is why they are called "T" cells). Both cells are responsible for the weighty task of protecting the body from infection, but they work in different manners.

B-cells are part of the innate immune system response. The innate immune system is responsible for creating antibodies that your body then uses to deactivate viruses the next time you come into contact with the same virus. Essentially, special B cells in the blood and lymph detect the protein of VZV and immediately recognize it as a non-self cell. At this point, the body's plasma cells manufacture specific glycoproteins called antibodies. The types of antibodies produced depend upon the type of infection that is occurring. In response to VZV, the plasma B cells will produce copious amounts of IgG antibodies, also called immunoglobulin G. Antibodies are shaped like a Y, with a spot shaped like a specific antigen for VZV on one of the spokes of the Y.

After they are activated by the T-cells, antibodies are present in blood, lymph and other body fluids and cells constantly patrolling for a repeat of the invading antigen. When these antibodies come into contact with a specific antigen, the antigen fits perfectly in the antibody, which then sounds the general alarm. When it recognizes the antigen of an invading VZV, the antibodies will neutralize that virus, preventing further infection. Antigen recognizing proteins are also present on the surface of B-cells. When these receptors come into contact with VZV, they activate and begin producing even more antibodies while they initiate the complement cascade, which eventually leads to VZV being destroyed by other specialized types of blood cells called macrophages and polymorphonuclear leukocytes. Macrophages and PMN are capable of engulfing viruses and bacteria and dismantling them. They then use the proteins to create more antibodies.

This process takes some time, which explains why primary infection with VZV results in chicken pox the first time an individual is exposed, and also why one does not typically get chicken pox twice. Once the body knows what to look for through the use of the antibodies, it can quickly mount the attack required to suppress the disease. In fact, exposure to those with active VZV infection (chicken pox) can serve to better protect the individual by giving their immune system a quick boost when exposed. The second time one is exposed to VZV or when the VZV tried to come out of dormancy, the body is ready for it and suppresses the activity for years.

The cell-mediated immune response, controlled by the

T-cells, responds to VZV in a much different manner. T-cells are the soldiers of the immune system. They serve as generals and footmen, hunting down the virus and killing them one by one. There must be careful checks and balances in place to ensure that the cell-mediated response does not become out of control and begin attacking the body cells. In order to ensure that this does not happen, the T-cells are able to recognize self and non-self cells. The T-cells literally hunt down and kill the viruses by engulfing them or by killing the cells that house the viruses.

When chicken pox infection has been stopped by the immune system, remaining VZV cells retreat into the deep neuron bodies and remain there dormant until they are reactivated. Scientists do not fully understand why the virus goes into a phase of dormancy, or why the lymphocytes do not find the dormant viruses inside the cell and destroy them in situ. One possible reason is because the cells that VZV chooses are nerve cells, which are notoriously protected by the body because of their incredibly slow rate of growth. The immune system's cells cannot even go with nerve cells because of the risk of damage to them. VZV is reasonably protected against the body's natural defenses while in the confines of nervous tissue.

Regardless of the reasons why, the viruses are left dormant, the innate response and the cell-mediated immune response are perpetually on the ready for any invading VZV. When they sense that the body has been exposed again, they swing into delightfully fast action, boosting immunity, creating thousands more lymphocytes and preventing disease. These little boosters of immunity are likely responsible for suppressing shingles disease and preventing VZV from reactivating.

Some critics of the varicella vaccine claim that it wasn't until the vaccine became commonplace that individuals began getting shingles in higher numbers. If, indeed, the body's response to being exposed to children with natural chicken pox was to boost immunity and keep the dormant cells at bay, then certainly the chance that vaccine has increased adults' risk of getting shingles. Without that boost of immunity provided my regular exposure, the body might be less likely to be able to mount an adequate defense.

When the reactivation of the virus happens, as occurs in shingles disease, the body's defenses are low or poorly developed, though doctors do not fully understand why this is in all cases. Completely healthy people can sometimes have a shingles outbreak; doctors do not understand the mechanism by which this happens. In some cases, the reason is obvious—the immune system has been somehow affected. This can be the case with individuals with HIV/AIDS, cancer or who take immunosuppressant drugs such as steroids or chemotherapeutics. Doctors also have indicated that excessive stress, as happens with the death of a partner or close friend, or the stressors brought on by a long-term harmful situation can cause an outbreak as well. In short, anything that lowers the body's ability to fight off disease can cause VZV to be able to reactivate.

Once someone has shingles disease, the immune system begins to increase its workload by producing more antibodies and more T-cells to combat the virus. This increase in immune system cells serves to protect the person from getting shingle disease again in the near future. Because of this boost, individuals do not typically get shingles twice in a short period of time. The increase in immune system cells can continue for decades to come without the person even being aware of their amazing body.

Some viruses shift in their DNA as they replicate, similar to what happens with HIV. These viruses care very difficult for the immune system to catch up with because as they divide, they change into other, equally harmful, viruses. The varicella zoster virus fortunately does not. Scientists think that VZV is much more stable than other viruses or retroviruses. VZV's stability helps to make it vaccine-preventable and to allow scientists the time to develop functional anti-viral drugs that can help to lessen the severity or eliminate the disease completely.

History of Shingles Disease

Shingles has been prevalent throughout the annals of history, though sometimes its effects were not clearly distinguished from other diseases that affected the skin such as leprosy and small pox. In fact, a British scientist named Herbeden postulated that the small pox was just a different manifestation of the same virus that causes chicken pox. He noted that some people had a pox; some died and some didn't. Herbeden did not know then that it was two completely different viruses causing the two diseases. He suspected that individual constitution determined who lives and who dies.

It wasn't until 1892 that scientists began to suspect that two entirely different viruses were responsible for chicken pox (at that time called swine pox) and small pox. Osler, a British physician, noted that having one of the diseases (either small pox or chicken pox) did not provide immunity for the other disease. Thus, a dual agent theory was born. He began closely tracking those who had chicken pox and those who he suspected had small pox and observing the differences in the presentation of the disease. Even in the 17th century, doctors had noticed that viruses conferred immunity to contracting the same disease again. This is the primary manner in which vaccinations were created. Therefore, they decided that the two presentations of small pox and chicken pox were caused by different organisms.

Also in 1892, a Bucharest pediatrician, James Bokay, observed several patients who became ill with shingles after having been exposed to children with chicken pox. This is the first mention of shingles in the medical annals. While the new disease seems to be a different presentation, he began to suspect that there was a link between the two diseases. He posited that the two diseases were inextricably linked. While no method of truly identifying the causative agent was possible in the late 19th century, scientist continued to assert that the two presentations of chicken pox and shingles were connected.

In 1921, a microbiologist named Lipshutz noticed that the both shingles and chicken pox had similar histopathology; the infected tissue sample of an individual with shingles looked very similar to the sample from an individual with chicken pox. He closely studied several cases of chicken pox and shingles and noticed that the cells in the two samples were both changed in the same manner, even though the disease seemed different. In 1948, the advent of the electron microscope was able to affirmatively identify the virus that causes chicken pox and shingles were entirely identical.

Because the nature of varicella zoster virus was to only slightly affect children with what was considered to be a benign childhood disease, scientists and physicians paid only fleeting attention to the virus itself. This makes sense because other, much more deadly diseases were prevalent and seemingly untreatable. It wasn't until human life expectancy began to extend that physicians began to see more frequent incidences of shingles appearing in the general population, primarily in adults. Doctors also began to note that VZV caused serious issues for the fetuses of pregnant women, those who were immune-compromised and adults who had not previously been exposed to VZV. VZV was also responsible for many missed hours of school and work, and added burdens to the already overburdened medical system. This shift in perception about the danger associated with varicella drove the desire to discover methods of treatment.

Doctors began to suspect that population could benefit from a vaccine that might protect children from chicken pox while simultaneously protecting adults from getting shingles. Vaccines are discussed in a separate section. Carefully studying virology has resulted in knowledge about viruses that eventually contributed to their demise. Viruses are not alive, in the truest sense of the word; trying to kill a non-living thing is extremely difficult if not impossible. But, with enough study of the virus life cycle, antiviral drugs were developed as options for treating infection with VZV.

Populations at Risk

Anyone who has been infected with varicella zoster virus at some point in his or her life is at risk of developing shingles disease. After primary infection, the virus lay dormant in the nerve cells. This latent infection gives rise to shingles, the secondary presentation of the virus, in about 32% of adults over the age of 60 years old who have been infected with natural VZV. By 85 years old, that number become 50% who have been infected. Adults younger than 60 are not the typical age for infection, and children only very rarely get shingles. Some individuals, however, are more likely to get shingles disease than others:

- **Individuals older than 60 years old**—People who are more than 60 years old are more likely to get shingles disease than those who are younger. Doctors suspect that the reason for the increase in shingles disease in older people can be attributed to the reduced functioning of the immune system as humans grow older. The longer the average human lifespan becomes, the more frequent shingles disease is likely to become, with potentially multiple recurrences for a single person as the virus shifts from dormancy into activity.

- **Individuals who had chicken pox in their first year of life**—when babies get chicken pox, their immune systems are immature and are bolstered by their mother's innate immunities passed to them through the placenta, colostrum and breastfeeding. Babies don't often catch chicken pox because of these reasons, and if they do, it can be very dangerous. Because their cell-mediated immune response is not yet fully functioning, babies a year of age or younger might not have enough antibodies to protect them from shingles disease long into their adult lives. For this reason, people who had chicken pox at a very young age are more susceptible to shingles disease than other individuals.

- **Individuals with Cancer**—People with cancer are often taking chemotherapeutic agents or radiation treatments that can reduce the number of healthy, functioning white blood cells (leukocytes). Without adequate numbers of strong leukocytes protecting the body, VZV might reactivate and cause shingles disease.

- **Individuals with Human Immunodeficiency Virus**—People living with HIV/AIDS often have fewer number of a specific type of leukocyte called a T-cell. T-cells are responsible for cell-mediated immune response that helps to suppress the reactivation of VZV. When individuals have fewer T-cells than their healthy counterparts, VZV reactivation is more likely to occur.

- **Individuals who are taking immuno-suppressant drugs**—For individuals who are taking immunosuppressant drugs, the body's immune system is less effective than people who have a normally functioning immune system. People may take an immune-suppressant for a variety of health conditions, including Systemic Lupus Erythema, rheumatoid arthritis and other autoimmune diseases.

- **Individuals who have a donor organ or bone marrow**—With an organ transplant or bone marrow transplant, long-term treatment with immunosuppressant drugs typically follow. These immunosuppressant drugs suppress the immune system as described above.

While all of the above populations are at-risk of developing shingles disease, anyone who has been infected with VZV is at risk of having it reactivate and cause shingles. Other issues that may allow reactivation include being under extreme psychological stresses and exposure to toxins in the environment. Essentially, anything that might increase susceptibility to illness can increase the chance that VZV will be able to reactivate within the nerve cells.

Race also plays a factor in the likelihood that one might get the disease. Caucasian individuals are also more likely to get shingles than their counterparts of African descent, though both races have an equal chance of becoming infected with VZV. This suggests that natural immunity in the black races might extend past the natural immunity of those of the Caucasian race. Some studies have also indicated a familial history of shingles might increase one's risk of getting shingles, though the literature has conflicting opinion about family history's impact.

Symptoms of Shingles Disease

While a primary infection with varicella zoster virus results in chicken pox, which presents with easily identifiable lesions on the whole body and systemic illness, shingles disease does not necessarily present the same way in every person. All individuals who have shingles will get the characteristic blister-like rash that affects one side of the body, but not all have the sensations that lead up to the rash and because the rash is not all over the body, it can be mistaken for other issues.

As the virus migrates down the nerve into the affected dermatome, the individual might begin experiencing tingling in the area that will eventually get shingles. The sensation might also be sensitivity, as though the area has been hurt or burned. Sometimes people experience heightened sensitivity to touch, water and even air in the regions that will be affected by VZV. Within a week, the sensation of tingling, itching or burning segues into a series of small, painful blisters that form in a cluster.

Other, more systemic issues also are associated with shingles disease. These symptoms can include fever, body aches, headache and general malaise. Often, it is these systemic symptoms that send people to the physician where they are often told that they likely have a viral illness that will not respond to medication. Most physicians will not recognize shingles before the trademark blistering rash occurs. While the cause is, indeed, viral in nature, there is a treatment for shingles disease.

The blisters range in amount of pain and type of pain experienced by the individual. Some people express that their pain is mild and primarily related to itching. Others describe intense pain that cannot be alleviated with analgesics. Some indicate that the slightest breeze will send them into horrific bouts of pain. The blisters sometime grow into a swath across the back or become inflamed like a burn. Usually, the affected region is in the torso, often on the back, but shingles can be anywhere on the body, including the scalp and the tip of the nose.

Individuals with shingles often describe their rash as being excruciating and describing it as unrelenting and not alleviated by anything at all. Some affected individuals express that they cannot place clothing or sheets or blankets on the rash, while still others state that even water from the shower feels as though their skin is on fire. This extreme pain requires treatment to alleviate the discomfort.

Most shingle disease blisters are located on only one side of the body, typically the torso or the back. Some people, particularly those whose reactivation has occurred from the trigeminal nerve, get herpes zoster opthalmicus, which causes conjunctivitis and other eye issues. If not properly treated, herpes zoster opthalmicus can progress into devastating damage in the eye. These serious complications of shingles are discussed further in a later section.

Shingles is also associated with a longer lasting form of pain called post-herpetic neuralgia, which are pain sensations that remain after the rash has resolved. Doctors suspect that the neuralgia is cause by the mechanism by which VZV travels—through the nerves that signal pain. Treatments for neuralgia range from analgesics, anticonvulsants, antivirals and anti-depressants.

The blisters continue for approximately three to four weeks and during that time, the blisters change from round and fluid-filled to crusty and dry. There may be a considerable amount of itching associated with the healing process. The pain of the blisters does not necessarily change as they progress from fluid-filed to crusty, but the systemic symptoms should feel better within two to three days. Until the blisters become dry, the infection is considered active and can be communicated to others. Taking care to cover the blisters or the rash is crucial in preventing the spread to non-immune people.

Contagiousness of Shingles

Like other viruses in the Herpesviridae family, varicella zoster virus is contagious for the period of time when the outbreak is occurring. The blister-like rash that happens in the active phase of shingles contains fluids that harbor the virus. The virus sheds in this manner and while people who touch the blisters will not get shingles, they are at risk of contracting VZV if they had not yet been exposed. Essentially, shingles is not contagious, but the virus that causes shingles is. If one contracts the disease from an individual with shingles, he or she will likely present with chicken pox, which is typically not dangerous for children. If an adult contracts chicken pox, the severity of the illness increases. If the exposed person is a VZV-free adult, there is the risk of serious complications.

For adults, in the US, it is unlikely that VZV exposure did not occur in childhood. But, as the incidence of natural chicken pox infection drops due to the presence of a vaccine for VZV, the chances of previous exposure will drop, and more people will be non-immune to the virus unless they become vaccinated. Further advancements in VZV vaccines and boosters can help prevent the incidence of shingles and VZV transmission, but caution remains important while in the intermediate period between partial vaccination coverage and full coverage for the public.

While chicken pox remains a relatively mild childhood disease and most children are vaccinated for varicella, there are some individuals who should not be exposed to shingles. These individuals include:

- **Children under the age of 1**—Children who are under the age of one year old have not been vaccinated against varicella and are at risk of not only contracting the disease, but passing the VZV to other children and adults. In addition, children with chicken pox can sometimes come into contact with people for whom shingles might be likely.

- **Pregnant Women**—Pregnant women who are exposed for the first time and contract varicella zoster virus can pass the infection on to their fetus, which can potentially complicate the baby's health. Pregnant women who have had chicken pox in the past are not in danger of contracting chicken pox because they already have it in the cells.

- **People with HIV/AIDS**—Individuals with shingles should be especially cautious of exposing their shingles rash to anyone who may have HIV/AIDS. Due to the nature of HIV, the important aspects of their immune systems, namely T-cells, can be severely compromised. Without the important T-cells, the body has an ineffective ability to prevent reactivation of VZV.

- **People with other preexisting conditions**—Conditions that are considered fairly well controlled can have a difficult time with shingles if they have an outbreak. Diabetes, as an example, can affect the blood flow to the extremities, which can cause complications for people with shingles.

- **Individuals with cancer**—Cancer victims are also likely to have a suppressed immune system. Chemotherapeutic agents, steroids and radiation can often change the composition of the blood cells constituents. If lymphocyte counts are lower than is typical, exposure to chicken pox or shingles can sometimes cause reactivation of the VZV residing dormant in the body.

While caution is indicated when one has shingles blisters for the sake of those around him or her who might not be vaccinated or naturally immune, there is also the risk of being the infected person being exposed to bacteria that might cause an opportunistic infection. The breaks in the skin, which is the most effective aspect of the immune system, can create the potential for dangerous bacteria that can cause severe infection or other complications. In the case of secondary bacterial infection, there is a risk that the infection could be with one of the types of bacteria that are resistant to treatment with antibiotics. Methicillin-resistant Staphylococcus aureus (MRSA) is a very real concern when one has exposed under layers of the skin and might require hospitalization for treatment with powerful intravenous antibiotics.

Special Case:

Pregnancy and Shingles Disease

For a woman who has had chicken pox in the past, shingles does not pose any additional risk than not being pregnant. Most women of childbearing age have been exposed to chicken pox in the past and so have natural immunity. For women who did not become exposed or have chicken pox as a child should consider having the chicken pox vaccine to prevent primary infection while pregnant. Some women do arrive at pregnancy without having had chicken pox or the vaccine, and shingles exposure for these women is very dangerous for the woman and her baby.

If the contagious person is in a household with someone who is pregnant and not immune to VZV (has not ever had the disease), extra special care should be taken to not expose the pregnant woman to VZV. Women cannot protect themselves with the chicken pox vaccine during pregnancy because it is not safe, so the only option for prevention is to avoid those who are contagious. While a natural immunity to VZV can protect the mother and the fetus, a primary infection with VZV during pregnancy can have catastrophic consequences. Through exposure through the placenta, the fetus is at risk of contracting VZV, but with a fledgling immune system, he or she is not capable of mounting an adequate defense to the disease.

If exposed in a first or second trimester pregnancy, congenital varicella syndrome has a very slight chance of happening. Congenital varicella syndrome causes some babies (0.4% to 2.0% of babies) to be born with issues with the limbs, eyes or brains. In some cases, the baby can be born with physical scarring on the skin. The baby will not have natural immunity because of this congenital infection with VZV. If exposed at term and just before the baby is due to be born, neonates may develop chicken pox immediately after birth. Chicken pox in a very small infant carries with it a death rate of 30%. If a pregnant woman becomes exposed and she does not know her immunity status, she should speak to her midwife or obstetrician immediately for advice about VZV infection.

Complications from Shingles

Shingles typically is considered to be a fairly benign, though painful disease. In the majority of cases, all is resolved within four to five weeks. Most cases of shingles disease resolve without any special treatment or concern. For all affected individuals, however, this is not the case. A number of possible complications for shingles can occur, some of which can be life threatening. The incidence of complications for shingles disease increases with the following risk factors: age, immune-compromised state, diabetes, cancer and HIV/AIDS. The following are the most frequently occurring complications of shingle disease and the rate of the occurrence of the complication:

- **Post-herpetic neuralgia (10-70%)**—Post-herpetic neuralgia is the most common complication of shingles disease. It is characterized by a continuation of pain sensation even after the shingles rash has resolved. For some people, post-herpetic neuralgia is completely debilitating; some of those affected by it are unable to engage in typical daily tasks. The symptoms of post-herpetic neuralgia include moderate to severe pain that continues for more than a month after the shingles disease has resolved and being very sensitive to pain and temperature. The populations that are at an increased risk for developing post-herpetic neuralgia include individuals who are older than 60 years of age,

26

women who have shingles disease, and individuals with a very advanced or difficult case of shingles disease.

Affected individuals describe the pain a variety of manners. The pain can be mild but chronic, very severe, stabbing, aching and feeling like an electric shock. Treatment for post-herpetic neuralgia can be a tricky prospect because this type of pain does not respond well to traditional approaches. If analgesics are effective, then options include ibuprofen, aspirin and acetaminophen. Sometimes, however, one might need narcotic pain management to control the symptoms of post-herpetic neuralgia. Options for narcotic pain control include oxycodone, codeine and other opiate prescriptions.

Other medications can also be effective. Some tricyclic antidepressants such as amitriptyline can help individuals to manage the pain because of the way that these medications affect the neurotransmitters, dopamine and serotonin, in the brain. Both dopamine and serotonin levels affect the way the body interprets pain sensations. There are several antidepressants that have a similar effect in the body and if a patient cannot tolerate one, physicians can try a different approach. Antidepressants can take up to two weeks for full effectiveness. Individuals who opt for this treatment option should be patient and not abandon the attempt because the medicine does take some time for full effectiveness.

In addition, some anticonvulsants can help

27

people manage the pain of post-herpetic neuralgia due to both their sedation effects and the manner with which the anticonvulsants affect the central nervous system's interpretation of pain. Phentoin is often prescribed, and carbamazepine has a particularly helpful effect on pain that is described as stabbing, sharp pain. Lamotrigine is especially effective on the sensation of burning and severe pain. Anticonvulsants can have a strong depressant effect on the central nervous system, which can make one excessively sleepy. Individuals who take anticonvulsants need to take care when operating cars or other machinery.

Some people find that non-traditional means of relief are in order for their post-herpetic neuralgia. Options for non-traditional pain management include heat and cold therapy, relaxation techniques such as yoga or controlled breathing patterns, and transcutaneous electrical nerve stimulation or TENS.

In 2010, a new option emerged for pain relief from post-herpetic neuralgia. A capsaicin patch that is applied for an extended period of time (one hour) can provide up to three months of relief. The treatment is quite expensive and ranges from $675 to $1,350 for a doctor's office treatment. As new options come available, the price for this patch is expected to reduce in price.

- **Bacterial skin infection (2.3%)**—Because the skin becomes broken in the normal course of shingles disease, exposure to bacteria can cause secondary skin infections. Typically, the skin protects the body against invasion of bacteria, and some bacteria even live on the skin's surface harmlessly. Bacteria that are common culprits include *Streptococcus* and *Staphylococcus*, which when introduced into broken skin can thrive and create an infection. An infection with *Staphylococcus aureus* can result in a hospital stay in isolation due to the incredibly virulent aspect of that bacteria and because it is resistant to antibiotics.

The bacterial infection can be challenging to identify in its earliest stages among a shingles outbreak because a first sign of infection is redness, which is already present. If the infection is not treated quickly, it can progress into a systemic infection that spreads through the bloodstream. Systemic infections can lead to severe symptoms and sepsis. Bacterial skin infections must be treated with antibiotic ointments that are perfectly suited for the specific bacteria. To determine the bacteria that have caused the infection, some doctors will require a culture of the area. If the infection has become systemic, it may require oral antibiotics to prevent further infection.

- **Eye Infection (1.6%)**—Eye infection occurs when the face or eye is the dermatome affected by the shingles disease. Moving from the trigeminal nerve into the skin on the face, VZV infection creates the same sensations as in the larger dermatomes. Eye infection, often called conjunctivitis, is redness and swelling of the conjunctiva of the eye. Because a virus causes it, there is no effective antibiotic drop available that can treat the eye infection. If a secondary infection occurs, the secondary bacterial infection can be treated with antibiotics for the eyes. Typically, it resolves on its own.

- **Neuropathy** (0.9%)—Neuropathy is generalized pain and paralysis in the muscles or connective tissue affected by VZV. After a bout with shingles some people report that they no longer have the ability to move an area of their body. Because neuropathy is essentially nerve damage, recovery takes quite a long time, but a full recovery can be expected.

- **Meningitis** (0.5%)—Meningitis is the inflammation of the tissue surrounding the brain. This complication can happen during shingles disease when the virus targets areas near the brain. This extremely dangerous complication can be accompanied by extreme head pain, fever, nausea and the inability to bend the chin to the chest. Viral meningitis cannot be treated with antibiotics, so treatment is largely palliative in nature. In some cases, anti-virals can be helpful in shortening the duration of the disease.

- **Herpes zoster opthalmicus** (0.2%)—This complication of shingles disease occurs when VZV moves from the trigeminal nerve into the optic nerve, which affects the eyes. Herpes zoster opthalmicus (HZO) begins in the same manner as typical shingles disease with general flu-type feelings. In about 60% of cases, the same pain, burning and heightened sensation accompanies HZO. About a week after symptoms begin, a rash of fluid-filled blisters breaks out across the forehead and on to the eyelids.

HZO continues in the same manner as shingles disease, with the blisters eventually bursting and then forming a crust, at which point the outbreak is no longer contagious. Unlike other types of shingles, HZO can be present for much longer. It can also lead to scarring and changes in the color of the skin permanently.

If the HZO appears on or around the nose (called Hutchinson Sign), the individual has a high chance of having damage to his or her cornea. Blisters that congregate around the nose signal that the nasocillary nerve is involved, which is the same nerve that innervates the cornea. This type of HZO is very dangerous because it changes the cornea of the affected eye. HZO that has affected the cornea may lead to a condition called keratitis, which is the inflammation of the cornea. Keratitis can be categorized based upon the region that is affected, and is extremely painful. To fully resolve, keratitis can take between a couple of days and a year.

Herpes zoster opthalmicus responds well to anti-viral medications including acyclovir, which can shorten the duration of the symptoms. Other medications that can help are corticosteroids, which can reduce the inflammation and analgesics to reduce the sensation of pain.

- **Disseminated varicella zoster virus**—In very rare and extreme cases, VZV can spread to other organs including the liver and lungs. Once VZV has been disseminated in the body, the affected organ becomes unable to maintain its workload. This very serious complication occurs mainly in people who have an immune system deficiency because of illness or medications. It is common in HIV/AIDS patients. This is a life threatening complication of shingles disease and usually only occurs with co-morbidities such as HIV/AIDS or severe immune-compromised status.

The majority of these complications occur most frequently in the special populations that are immune-compromised in some manner. HIV/AIDS patients, cancer patients, elderly people and transplant recipients are the most likely to have these complications. While all of these complications are fairly rare in people who have shingles disease, the possibility exists that one might require advanced treatment for these issues. Seeking out a healthcare practitioner is vital in these cases to adequately determine what the proper diagnosis and treatment for shingles disease might be.

Diagnosis of Shingles

When one suspects that he or she might have shingles disease, a trip to his or her primary care physician should be at the top of the to-do list. While shingles appears to be a dermatological disorder, there is no compelling reason to see a dermatologist unless the patient is referred to one by his or her primary care physician. Sometimes a trip to the dermatologist does seem to make sense. Because shingles is a fairly common disease, primary care doctors are generally well prepared to handle the diagnosis.

Most healthcare practitioners will immediately recognize the signs and symptoms of shingles disease. Upon presentation at the emergency room or the primary care facility, physicians will be able to spot the telltale-blistering rash accompanied by pain and flu-like symptoms. On some occasions, particularly early in the disease presentation, it can be difficult to distinguish shingles disease from other viral illnesses. Once the rash breaks out, however, doctors can spot the disease easily. Most patients state that the reason they went to the doctor to begin with is because they were experiencing pain. They go into the ER or their doctor's office only because they wish to get pain relief. They are not sure what is wrong, but they know it is painful.

The first step to determining whether or not one has shingles is to rule out other diseases that resemble shingles. These include bacterial infection of the skin, infection with herpes simplex, and other skin-related disorders. Because these other conditions have different treatment options than shingles disease, it is vital that the proper diagnosis is made. To assist the physician in the proper diagnosis, the following tests are available to determine the cause of the rash:

- **Culture of the rash**—If the doctor suspects that the rash could be related to herpes simplex virus, it might be necessary to culture a sample of the virus from either the rash or from cerebrospinal fluid. Taking a sample from the rash is a simple procedure that involves using a cotton swab to gently scrape the blisters to remove some of the virus. Taking a sample of cerebrospinal fluid requires an invasive test called a lumbar puncture where a doctor carefully guides a needle aspirator into the spinal column to withdrawn fluid. Doctors then culture the sample from either source in a specially prepared growing medium to see what virus develops. This process can take up to two weeks for accurate results. This test, while conclusive, can take valuable time that could be used in treatment for shingles.

- **Immunofluorescence Assay Test**—Because it is both less expensive and faster than a culture, most physicians will use the immunofluorescence assay test to determine whether or not the infection is VZV. This test requires a sample as well, which is then subjected to immunofluorescence, or ultraviolet light waves. The antibodies produced in the normal course of shingles disease will then appear when laboratory specialists look at the sample through a microscope. Test results are back within several days.

- **Polymerase Chain Reaction (PCR)**—PCR is a useful technique when it is necessary to determine whether or not shingles disease has become disseminated in the body. Samples from viruses (even a broken fragment) is replicated over and over until there is enough identifiable virus available to make a determination about what is causing the infection. This is an extremely expensive, but unfailingly accurate method of determining the cause of the infection. With advances in new technology, PCR might become the gold standard in the identification of shingles and other diseases.

The physician will likely also order a series of blood tests that can determine whether or not the infection is viral or bacterial, but these blood tests are also used to determine the immune status of the individual with shingles disease. This vital step provides doctors with a good baseline result for the complete blood county—the levels of leukocytes and erythrocytes that are currently circulating in the blood. Because shingles disease often happens when individuals have other systemic issues and diseases, taking blood gives doctors an up-close look at how efficiently the body currently functions. Doctors might choose to do a number of panels to determine how the body systems are functioning including liver, thyroid and kidney panels.

The first blood test that physicians will likely perform is the complement-fixation test (CFT). CFT looks at the body's immune response to shingles to determine whether or it is has begun the process of using the complement system to bind antigens from the shingles disease. Specifically, this test looks at the levels of bound antibodies and to which antigens they have bound. It tests for levels of IgG in the blood. This test can adequately determine whether or not the immune system has the ability to mount an adequate defense to the VZV reactivation. It can be difficult to tell the difference between herpes simplex and varicella with a CFT test.

Next, doctors may test for VZV antigens in the blood through enzyme immunoassay (EIA) or radioimmunoassay (RIA) testing. This test will positively identify current or previous infection with VZV through looking at IgG antibodies. IgG antibodies are created by specialized B cells called plasma cells, and they indicate that the secondary innate response has been engaged by the innate immune system. While this is a sensitive test, there may be some limitations in the information provided back to the physician. For example, if co-infection with herpes simplex virus is present in the individual, this test might produce a "false" positive. This test is best used in conjunction with other tests.

Also, doctors will likely test the individual for a complete blood count, which indicates the levels of specific components of the blood including all types of leukocytes, erythrocytes and other tests as necessary. Blood tests provide physicians with enough background information to help make the diagnosis of shingles disease while simultaneously giving information about the general state of individual health. All of these tests can lead to a diagnosis and a plan for treatment.

Treating Shingles

After diagnosis, the doctor and the patient will develop a treatment plan to help counteract the shingles infection. The treatment plan has several goals and will serve to guide both the patient and the doctor along the path to recovery. Treatment for shingles functions to reduce the sensations of pain, provide accelerated healing for the blistering rash, prevent transmission to others, and to reduce the general bodily discomfort associated with shingles disease. Unfortunately, treatment for shingles is rarely a singular approach that works perfectly for each person with shingles. The treatment is highly individualized and depends greatly on the health status of the person with shingles, the severity of the disease and the available resources to treat the illness.

Individuals with shingles disease often want the first priority to be the mitigation of their pain sensations. Sometimes an over-the-counter (OTC) analgesic preparation can provide enough relief to the person with shingles so that stronger prescription-only medication need not be used. OTC analgesics include acetaminophen, aspirin and ibuprofen. Aspirin should never be given to children due to the small risk of Reye's Syndrome, though children rarely will get shingles disease. If these medications do not work, then doctors might prescribe a stronger, narcotic analgesic that combines aspirin or acetaminophen with medications such as oxycodone, hydrocodone or codeine. Narcotic pain relievers can cause drowsiness or sedation, so the patient must be cautious when engaging in work that might require full alertness or concentration. In addition, narcotic pain relievers can cause dependency and should not be taken long term. They are for short term use only.

Another common method of treating shingles disease includes antiviral medications. Antivirals come with different mechanisms of action. All antivirals act to shorten the duration of the attack and contagion of the rash. Antivirals do not kill VZV, but rather they cause the virus to stop replicating, reducing the level of the virus in the body. Antivirals can reduce the sensation of pain, accelerate the healing of the blisters and rash, reduce itching and reduce the risk of developing post-herpetic neuralgia. But, antivirals do not cure shingles disease.

The most popular oral antiviral is part of the drug class called nucleoside analogues. Nucleoside analogues prevent the virus from using an important nucleoside called guanosine. Guanosine is an important part of VZV's ability to replicate itself. Nucleoside analogues are shaped similarly to guanosine, but the nucleoside analogues do not provide the virus with the chemicals that will allow them to replicate. When the virus tries to use the nucleoside analogues instead of guanosine, the replication process stops. The life cycle of the virus is inhibited, but the actual virus is not destroyed.

Nucleoside analogues that doctors usually prescribe include acyclovir, famciclovir, and valacyclovir. All three of these drugs function in the same way in the body, and all are approved for shingles disease. Acyclovir requires that the individual take the drug five times per day, which can be very difficult to adhere to for the patient. The other two drugs, famciclovir and valacyclovir, require doses every 12 hours, which can be much easier for the patient to adhere to.

Famciclovir and valacyclovir both break down into acyclovir when introduced into the body, and so all are the same nucleoside analogue.

Treatment using nucleoside analogues should be started within 72 hours of an outbreak of shingles, though if one doesn't begin taking it until after that, it can still be helpful in reducing pain and discomfort and will still somewhat speed healing. While most people with shingles disease can recover without the use of antivirals, the CDC recommends that certain populations of people take antivirals to reduce the chance of a complication from shingles disease. These populations include the elderly, individuals with underlying health conditions such as HIV or diabetes, and individuals who may develop herpes zoster opthalmicus.

Side effects for nucleoside analogue treatment can be irritating, but the benefit to the drugs can outweigh the risks of using them. Rash, headache, nausea and vomiting, extreme fatigue and tremors can accompany the use of any of the nucleoside analogues. In some cases, the side effects of taking antivirals can include kidney damage and blood clots particularly in people with existing immune issues such as HIV or AIDS. Many think that the risk to the nucleoside analogues are not a concern.

Other antivirals include foscavir and brivudin. Foscavir is a pyrophosphate analogue, which means that it is shaped similarly to pyrophosphate. The VZV virus uses pyrophosphate as part of its replication cycle. Foscavir can only be administered intravenously and only in the case of drug-resistance to acyclovir. Foscavir has major side effects including fever, nausea, and ulcers. Brivudin is an antiviral that shows great promise and has the benefit of only needing to take it one time per day, but currently it is not available in the United States.

Some doctors wish to prescribe corticosteroids. These drugs provide anti-inflammatory effects that can help with swelling, redness and excessive inflammation. Prednisolone or prednisone are examples of corticosteroids. Typically, they are prescribed for the first couple of weeks only because their effect quickly wanes. Usually they are taken along with a nucleoside analogue. While corticosteroids are often prescribed, studies indicate that they have questionable benefit to those with shingles. They do not in any way prevent shingles from occurring, nor do they mitigate the chances that one might get post-herpetic neuralgia. While it was commonplace to prescribe corticosteroids for shingles in the past, this practice is quickly becoming old-fashioned. Corticosteroids can be taken orally or they can be injected or intravenous. Side effects to corticosteroids include irritability, weight gain and swelling.

For more localized pain relief, doctors can prescribe a lidocaine patch that provides a topical anesthetic that will numb the affected area. The patches provide approximately 300 mg of lidocaine per patch. Three patches at once can be applied if a larger area needs to be covered. The patches are not to be applied if the area still is covered in blisters, but once the blisters disappear, the patches can provide almost immediate, complete relief to the area for many hours at a time. Lidocaine patches are a great option for pain relief, particularly if the individual experiences post-herpetic neuralgia.

Treatment for shingles may include all of the above treatment or none of it. The doctor will make a decision on the treatment needed and the safety associated with it. Many people choose to forgo medications in favor of treating their shingles at home or with alternative modalities. Before embarking on a natural course of treatment, be sure to check with the doctor to ensure that it is a safe prospect.

Home and Alternative Treatments

For individuals who have a mild form of shingles disease that does not require the use of prescription medication or those who choose not to seek out medical treatment, there are some at-home remedies that can help alleviate the discomfort of shingles disease. Alternative treatments have also been proved to be marginally helpful in reducing the severity of the disease as well. Please consult a physician before using any alternative modality especially if prescription medication has been prescribed because of the potential for interactions.

One of the simplest options for reducing the pain of shingles disease is to use cold therapy. This can be performed in several ways. First, using a commercially prepared instant cold pack can be helpful. These are packaged and ready to use once your break the inner portion that provides the cold. Be sure that the instructions are followed carefully and that the packs are not applied to bare skin. Cold packs that are applied to bare skin can cause burning that can lead to infection.

A reusable cold pack is also exceptionally helpful. These gel-filled bags can be placed in the freezer for several hours to freeze; once they are cold enough, they can be applied to the affected area of the skin. Wrapping the reusable cold pack in a towel or a pillowcase can help protect the sensitive skin. If cold does seem to alleviate some of the pain, taking a cool (not cold) bath can help to soother the rash as well. Using some well-ground oatmeal, or a commercially prepared oatmeal soak, can help to make the skin feel supple and soft.

Nutritional supplementation can also help the body heal from shingles disease. Supplements can interact with medication, so if an individual is currently taking medication prescribed by a doctor, he or she should first consult a physician. The following supplements can be useful in treating shingles disease:

- **Adenosine monophosphate** (AMP)—AMP is a naturally occurring chemical and has shown promise in treating shingles based upon early studies. It is taken orally, intravenously or it can be injected via intramuscular injection. AMP has shown promise in helping to reduce pain in shingles disease. A study of individuals with shingles indicated that their blood serum levels of AMP were lower than is typical. As a result, supplementation with AMP can help bring those levels back to normal. The actual mechanism of action for AMP is not yet known, though studies indicate that there might be some benefit from supplementation with AMP. AMP is routinely used in hospitals to treat arrhythmia and other conditions. One study indicated an 88% pain relief rate after four weeks in individuals who were given an injection with AMP, compared with 43% who were given a placebo. Clearly, more studies need to be conducted, but evidence suggests some help for individuals supplementing with AMP.

- **Vitamin B6 and B12**—B6 and B12 are both essential vitamins for the body. B vitamins help the nerves in the body function properly in a healthy body. A deficiency in this group alone can cause neuralgia, or pain related to the nerves, even without the condition of shingles. Because nervous tissue harbors varicella zoster virus, which uses the nerves to move to the affected dermatomes, a deficiency in B vitamins can cause further issues in the nervous tissue. B12 typically is either given sublingually (under the tongue) or by injection by a licensed health care provider. B6 is taken orally.

- **Vitamin E**—Vitamin E is essential for the proper functioning of the skin. Vitamin E can also reduce the incidence of scarring and also help protect nerves from viral attack. Because the skin is affected in shingles disease, vitamin E can prove an invaluable resource. Some studies have found that taking vitamin E during a shingles attack can help reduce pain and inflammation. While more studies are needed to confirm this, taking a vitamin E supplement can be beneficial in the fight against shingles. Because vitamin E is a fat-soluble vitamin, it can be toxic in large doses. Be sure to verify the dose before taking excessive amount of vitamin E.

- **L-lysine**—L-lysine, an essential amino acid, cannot be manufactured in the body; it must be either obtained through nutrition or supplementation. While some people take this amino acid as a well-known way of preventing herpes outbreaks, the way l-lysine works in the body can help to protect against shingles as well. It interferes with the viral life cycle and can help reduce the severity of the shingles outbreak. L-lysine is available as a oral tablet.

Some foods are also rich in lysine such as legumes, Brewer's yeast, cheese, meat and fish.

Acupuncture can also be helpful in treating the pain associated with shingles. A licensed acupuncture physician can apply sterile acupuncture needles in areas of the body to help reduce the pain of shingles. Acupuncture physicians (APs) are trained in identifying the levels of a force called qi in the body. If there is a deficiency of qi in one part of the body, the application of an acupuncture needle or several needles can help to open the blockage of qi. While oriental medicine is not often practiced in certain regions of the US, there are many studies that indicate the usefulness and effectiveness of visiting with an AP. APs are also able to use the technique of moxibustion, which is the practice of burning certain herbs around the areas of the body that are affected by shingles. Many claim that mugwort moxibustion is especially helpful in relieving pain associated with shingles.

In addition to cold therapy, supplementation and acupuncture, herbal preparations can also be useful in treating shingles disease. Herbal medicine can be considered by some to be questionable in efficacy and safety, but many of the medicines used by physicians today were developed using herbal preparations. Herbs, unfortunately, are often not tested for safety and effectiveness because research studies are very expensive and herbs are common use products. There is often little recent, empirical evidence that herbs make much of a difference, but centuries of healers have used herbal preparations to resolve issues in the body. Because herbs are powerful substances and can cause interactions with other drugs, individuals who are considering taking herbs should speak to their physicians before beginning any herbal therapy. The following herbs are considered helpful for shingles disease:

- **Cayenne Pepper** (*Capsicum frutescens*)—Cayenne, a powerful herb, has been used for many years for a variety of health conditions. Capsaicin, a major constituent of cayenne, is harvested to use in commercially prepared creams and lotions to treat the pain of arthritis and other painful conditions. Cayenne is used in newly developed prescription strength applications that can provide relief for up to three months. Supplementation for cayenne can be taken orally or in a cream or lotion to apply externally. Over-the-counter preparations are available for external use.

- **Chamomile Flower** (*Matricaria recutita*)—Chamomile has long been used in teas and tinctures for its mild sedation effects. Chamomile is mild enough that even children's preparations contain it. While its effects have not been studied for shingles, the soothing quality to chamomile makes it an exceptional choice for a liniment or a cream to apply externally. In addition, chamomile might provide some anti-inflammatory relief if taken as a supplement in teas or tinctures.

- **Licorice Root (*Glycyrrhiza glabra*)**—Licorice's main constituent is glycyrrhizin, which in some studied has shown promise in stopping VZV replication. Licorice has long been used as a topical treatment for shingles, and there may be some benefit to its ingestion as well. Licorice root can also be used as an anti-depressant similar in type to St. John's Wort. In some studies, licorice root was shown to increase the body's amount of interferon, which is a chemical mediator that is used by the immune system cells to stop the growth of viruses. In this manner, licorice root might be a beneficial addition to a herbal regimen during shingles outbreaks. It is also well documented that licorice has been shown to interact with prescription medications, so a physician should be aware before an individual with shingles takes licorice. Licorice root can also increase blood pressure, so those with hypertension should be cautious in taking this herb.

Homeopathy also can be used in the treatment of shingles, though its effectiveness is mainly supported by anecdotal or observational data. Homeopathy involves the ingestion of highly diluted material that is known to cause the symptom that is being treated. Preparations are assigned based upon very specific symptoms. An individual should see a homeopath before taking any remedies, so that he or she can take a full physical and recording of symptoms. Homeopathy is highly controversial, though there has been no documented harm of using its principles. In shingles, the following herbs are considered to be helpful:

- **Rhus toxicodendron**—This remedy is indicated for unrelenting itching as well as pain that seems to feel better when touched.

- **Lachesis**—Individuals use this remedy for a rash that is dark in color and located on the left side only.

- **Arsenicum**—This remedy relieves a sensation of burning that seems to be better when one applies heat to the skin, and is also used for feverish symptoms.

- **Mezereum**—This remedy is primarily used by people who become cold easily and is used to treat stabbing, burning pains associated with shingles.

- **Ranunclus bolbosus**—Individuals who have a rash on their back or their chest and for whom the pain seems to be untouchable and worse with movement.

Homeopathy was postulated in the 1800s and has been used since, though in the US its use is not a common complementary medicine option. While the theory seems to be contradictory to current scientific findings, many report quite good results while using remedies. Some claim that the positive effects of homeopathy are only placebo effects, but for one suffering from shingles disease, any possible relief would be welcome.

An additional option for alternative treatments is focusing on the body-mind connection. Because shingles is often caused by excessive stress, which can weaken the immune system response, reducing stress in one's life can have a positive effect. Meditation, focused breathing, yoga and progressively relaxing one's muscles has been shown to have a positive effect on calming the mind, which in turn can help reduce pain. There are even some reports that hypnosis can be helpful in reducing the sensation of pain. Some doctors suggest taking time off of work and avoid stressful situations that might increase the severity of the illness.

Regardless of the track one takes with treatment, there are numerous options available for at-home and complementary medical care. What works for one may not transfer and work for another, so a piecemeal approach might be in order. A doctor's approval for alternative modalities might be required for some individuals, particularly if one is in the high-risk category due to immune system issues; has underlying medical issues such as HIV, diabetes or cancer; or has an extremely complicated shingles infection.

Vaccination for Shingles Disease

Along with treatment, protection from shingles can result from a vaccine, called Zostavax. Zostavax provides protection from shingles by boosting the body's preexisting antibodies so that one's own immune system will continue to keep the virus in dormancy preventing the reactivation of the varicella zoster virus. Before the varicella vaccine, adult exposure to children with the chicken pox performed this function for adults—exposure to the virus caused a boost in immune function that seemed to keep the virus at bay. Without this periodic boost, one's own immune system may not be enough to prevent a shingles outbreak.

Critics of the varicella and shingles vaccine claim that without the varicella vaccine effectively decreasing the incidence of naturally acquired varicella, while simultaneously raising the incidence of shingles outbreaks. They further claim that without the varicella vaccine the rates of shingles outbreaks would not indicate a vaccine. While some studies do support the notion that the shingles rates have greatly increased in the years following the vaccine's widespread use, other studies indicate that the increase is negligible.

Zostavax is prepared by using human cells to culture a form of varicella zoster virus that is both live and attenuated. This means that the virus has not been killed and its constituent parts used, but rather it has been altered slightly so that its effects in the body are not as virulent. The live, attenuated virus is injected subcutaneously (under the skin). From there, the body's immune system begins to work producing antibodies to fight the virus, which will not cause disease because of its attenuated status. The immune response follows the same process as outlined in a previous section of this work, with B and T cells acting to protect the body from harm.

Scientists developed Zostavax as a means to help prevent serious shingles disease in those for whom a shingles outbreak can be dangerous. Shingles has become more prevalent in the years since the varicella vaccine. Merck drug manufacturers completed the development of a shingles vaccine in 2005 and entered investigational status for approval. After six years, Merck's vaccine was approved; the FDA then began to recommend the vaccine for adults aged 60 years and older. After a lukewarm reception by the elderly US population, the FDA expanded the public recommendation to include those ages 50-59. Side effects of Zostavax are few and included headache and irritation at the site of the injection.

Zostavax's safety and effectiveness was observed in a three-year study involving 38,000 participants aged 60-80, half of whom were vaccinated and half who were given a placebo. The study supported the claim that individuals who were vaccinated had a 50% lower chance of getting shingles. While some studied did develop shingles, their illness was much less severe than expected. Bolstered by these results, another study was performed on 22,000 individuals ages 50-59 to determine the effects in a younger age bracket. This study indicated that people in this age bracket were 70% less likely to get shingles.

Regardless of its efficacy, Zostavax should not be given to certain members of the population because it is a vaccine that contains a live virus. Those who should not be given the injection of Zostavax are people who have immune system weaknesses or people who are in treatment for cancer, taking steroids for any reason, or have cancer in their lymphatic system, their bone or their blood. If an individual has HIV or AIDS, he or she should consult with a physician before getting the Zostavax shot. In addition, if one is allergic to gelatin or neomycin, he or she cannot receive the vaccine because they might be at risk of a severe allergic reaction.

Zostavax has had some issue getting support from doctors and patients alike. A primary reason that this vaccine has had a less than optimal reception is because Merck was initially unable to make enough vaccine to supply the entire country. Once the supply reached a reasonable level, patients had to deal with the cost of the vaccine, which in 2011 was more than $200. While not covered by all private health insurances, Medicare Part D covers Zostavax. Regardless, it can be difficult to store Zostavax in mobile clinics such as those at drug stores because it requires a freezer for storage. Expanding the market to include adults aged 50 to 59 years old will help create a demand for the vaccine and ideally protect more people.

Like all vaccines, there are those who will refuse to be vaccinated based upon personal reasons. These reasons include wariness about the safety of vaccines, especially new ones that have not been thoroughly tested over long term studies. In addition, some cite concern that the use of embryonic cells from the products of an abortion makes the vaccine run contrary to their religious principles. Still others feel that vaccines in general can cause autoimmune disorders or other chronic illnesses. Some people feel that a vaccine for the prevention of shingles is not worth the injection because shingles, while painful, is not life threatening and does not serve to cause any major lasting effects.

Zostavax has been proven to be safe with numerous clinical trials as well as targeted databases that look at the effectiveness of the vaccine versus the incidence of side effects. While it does contain a live virus, this is only dangerous in the case of an immune-compromised individual. While some will experiences headaches with the use of Zostavax, no other adverse side effects are yet appended to the prescribing information for physcians.

The US Vaccine Adverse Event Reporting System (VAERS) has established protocol to report the incidence of adverse events associated with both the varicella vaccine and the shingles vaccine. Over the course of many years, its data will be collated and condensed into an appropriate risk number so that individuals for whom the vaccine is an option can determine whether or not the risk outweighs the benefit to getting vaccinated for shingles.

Recurrence of Shingles

Because of the way varicella zoster virus functions within the body, getting shingles once may help protect against getting it a second time. When VZV becomes reactivated and moves through the nerves, the immune system mounts another response to the presence of the newly replicated viruses. The T-cells begin to attack the virus-infected cells, and the B-cells release newly manufactured antibodies.

While the individual is in the midst of the shingles outbreak, the body is working hard to contain the infection and encourage it into dormancy. Once the body is able to overcome the virus, and it re-enters dormancy in the dorsal ganglion or trigeminal nerve tissue, the virus returns to its latent state and ideally will stay that way for the remainder of the individual's life. Sometimes, however, an outbreak of shingles is not enough to keep the virus in its dormant state for the remainder of the lifespan.

A 2009 study, however, indicates that shingles may recur more often than physicians predicted previously. This study indicates that once an individual has had single outbreak of shingles disease, the rate of a subsequent outbreak is approximately 30%, which is the same chance of having a primary outbreak of shingles in the first place. The resulting data suggested that even people who have had shingles in the past get the vaccination for shingles. This study, funded by Merck, has been questioned because of the apparent conflict of interest. Other studies immediately signed up to look at chances of recurrence.

In June 2012, a large study of 6,000 cases of shingles with follow up indicated that the incidence of recurrence was much lower than indicated by the 2009 study. Out of 6,000 patients, fewer than 30 of the unvaccinated study participant had shingles recur a second time in the three years of the study. This gives the rate of remission of approximately 24 out of 10,000 individuals, as compared to 19 out of 10,000 in vaccinated population. This difference isn't considered to be statistically significant enough to warrant vaccination among people who have already had shingles. Therefore, there is no advantage to vaccinating people who have already had shingles because there is no more likelihood that they will benefit from the vaccine.

Recurrence is greater in those individuals who had a more difficult or painful time with their outbreak of shingles. If the shingles was painful enough to warrant the use of strong narcotics or require hospitalization, it may be more likely to recur. It is also more likely if the individual is immune-compromised or taking medication that makes him or her immune-compromised. Also, the likelihood of recurrence is proportional to the age of the patient. The older a patient is, the more likely they are to have a recurrence.

Unfortunately for some individuals, recurrence seems to happen more than twice. In fact, several reports of people experiencing what seems to be a frequent return to the blistering rash has scientists taking a second look at what some are calling chronic shingles. These individuals will sometimes get a small break between outbreaks, but then the burning and itching comes back with a vengeance a short time later. More investigation needs to occur to learn more about why these individuals are experiencing this phenomenon.

Individuals who have had shingles disease once know what to expect the second time around. In fact, there is some evidence that knowing what to expect can help reduce the length of the severity. If one remembers the feeling of tingling and burning of the previous outbreak, seeking out medical help early might contribute to a faster recovery time. Starting the antiviral medication and any other alternative modality as early as possible can help to shorten the duration of the disease.

Prognosis for Shingles Disease

When an individual has shingles, the prognosis is typically very straightforward. Approximately one week after shingles disease presents with fever, body aches and malaise, the blistery rash erupts on the aspect of the body that is affected by the VZV infection. The rash, which can be expected to be painful and blistery, will follow a course from raised and fluid-filled to open and crusty. While there might still be pain associated with the rash, once the crusty appearance has formed, the individual is no longer contagious to others. For the majority of individuals who have shingles, the rash is entirely gone within five weeks; the pain associated with the rash is likewise gone. There should be little to no scarring of the skin from the shingles outbreak.

Approximately one in five shingles sufferers will get a complication from the disease. Most will suffer from post-herpetic neuralgia and experience pain for weeks to months after the infection as subsided. Complications include secondary bacterial infection and eye involvement. In very rare cases, encephalitis and systemic viral infection can occur. Complications will increase the duration of the disease and may require additional treatment for the conditions. If herpes zoster opthalmicus occurs, it may take up to a year for the condition to resolve completely.

Some studies have indicated an increased risk of cancer following shingles disease. Individuals who have had shingles have a 1.8% risk of developing cancer in the first year following the shingles outbreak. The cancers most often represented included immune related cancers, blood cancers, and cancers of the lung, brain and cervix.   While those with non-blood related cancers had a normal disease progression, those who had blood cancer had a much lower survival rate than individuals who have never had shingles suffering from the same cancer. Brain cancer risk seems to be much higher than in individuals who did not have shingles. The study indicated that those who were hospitalized for shingles had the highest risk of cancer. The study corrected for cancers that were discovered while the person had active shingles because the cancer and the shingles, while coexisting, were not causative in nature. Scientists do not know why the link between cancer and shingles exists, but studies in the future will be likely to look at the connection and determine the reason and which causes which.

Epidemiology of Shingles Disease

Shingles occurs worldwide, with the lowest shingle rates in tropical regions. Transmission of varicella zoster virus, which causes shingles, occurs through the transmission of infected droplets or by direct contact with an infectious shingles rash. The droplets contain VZV with a sufficient viral load to cause infection. Despite centuries of documented occurrence, shingles is purely a human disease. It cannot be communicated to or contracted from animals. There is not one particular time of year that people can experience a shingles outbreak; cases occur all year long.

While the CDC does not require health department and private doctors to make notification about the disease, it does estimate that between 500,000 and 1 million people in the US have a shingles outbreak per year. In a lifetime, the average risk of having a shingles outbreak is about 32%, while increasing age increases the risk. By age 85, 50% of the US population will have had at least one shingles outbreak.

The varicella zoster virus is extremely contagious and will easily spread among families, school children and the workplace. Care should be taken to limit exposure if one knows that he or she has a contagious rash. Shingles, however, does not occur in epidemics and one cannot catch shingles from another individual with shingles. One can catch VZV and become infected if not already immune to it. No compelling evidence exists for a familial link for shingles outbreaks. A family history of shingles does not predispose one to getting shingles in their adulthood.

There is some reason to believe that the inclusion of the chicken pox vaccine in the routine vaccination schedule has led to a marked increase in shingles outbreaks. Scientists suspect that this is related to the decrease in chicken pox due to the vaccine has eliminated or reduced adult exposure to VZV, which means that adults have been losing that extra little boost of immunity provided by the exposure to the virus. Hospitalization costs for shingles have increased more than $700 million from 1996 to 2001. Other studies found that the incidence of shingles increased by an average of 90%. This increase in shingles led to the development of a shingles vaccine, which is now being marketed to those 50 years of age and older. As the children who had the vaccine begin to come into the range where shingles is typical, epidemiologist will be watching closely and wondering if their experiment has paid off.

Prevention of Shingles

Once an individual has contracted varicella zoster virus, it is in the body forever. While the primary infection causes chicken pox, the dormant virus can at any point shift into reactivation and cause shingles. Doctors suggest that there are some ways to help prevent shingles from occurring. Because scientists do not fully understand what makes VZV shift from dormancy to reactivation, there's not a sure way to prevent its occurrence without using the shingles vaccine.

The shingles vaccine is a one-time injection for individuals over 50 years old. Of course, the shingles vaccine has a high efficacy rate with few side effects; 55% fewer shingles outbreaks occur after having been vaccinated. Before the age of 50, however, the vaccine is not available, nor has it been tested or deemed appropriate for that age group. In addition, there was not much of a decline in people older than 85 years old who were vaccinated.

To prevent shingles from occurring, doctors recommend keeping the body healthy through nutrition and exercise. Be sure to consume adequate amounts of foods rich in antioxidants that can keep cells healthy deep within your body. Antioxidants prevent harmful free radicals from harming cells as they age. Maintain a health immune system by getting regular check-ups with a licensed physician. Some evidence suggests that eating a diet rich in L-lysine might help prevent outbreaks. Foods rich in L-lysine include fish, meats and eggs.

Regular exercise might play a part in keeping the mind and body as healthy as possible. People who regularly exercise have a lower incidence of stress-related illness, which might include shingles. While no research based study has been conducted, common sense tells us that when the mind and body are healthy and active, the immune system is likely to be working its hardest. Exercise also helps reduce the levels of stress hormones in the body, which might help the immune system stay at peak performance.

Regardless of the amount of work that one might invest in not getting shingles, there is no 100% way of ensuring that one can prevent it. In fact, not even the shingles vaccine claims 100% effectiveness. Even after getting the shingles vaccine, some people get shingles. Even after getting shingles and then the vaccine, some people get shingles again. It's not the fault of the individual who gets shingles, and there is truly nothing for certain that they could do to prevent the occurrence.

Because there is not a sure way to know who will and will not have a shingles outbreak, education is the key to prevention. Armed with enough knowledge about the expected course of the disease individuals can closely monitor themselves for any unusual sensation that might be shingles. Once he or she notices the burning, painful sensation, he or she might recognize it immediately as shingles and get treatment that might lessen the severity of the disease. Educational outreach can improve not only the duration of shingles, but the severity of it as well.

On the Horizon for Shingles

Despite the vast amounts of knowledge already known about VZV and its manifestation as shingles, many scientists feel that more study is necessary to fully understand not only the disease but the human immune system response. Studies are planned to develop a broader understanding of shingles and its implications for the healthcare system, the economy and individual health and wellness.

In the future, scientists will continue to monitor the incidence of shingles and any complications to which it might lead. Because shingles has not yet been declared to be "notifiable" by the CDC, keeping these records comes down to voluntary record-keeping at the local or state level. Some suggestions for keeping more accurate data on who gets shingles and where, include large open-access databases and surveys by states or counties about shingles outbreaks.

Scientists also want to ensure that the current recommended vaccine, Zostavax, maintains its level of protection over the course of many years. Currently, it seems that there may be some waning of protection over a twenty-year span. More studies are necessary to determine if protection continues to ebb or if it remains constant over the long term. Knowing this information might help inform policy about vaccine schedules and may result in the inclusion of a Zostavax booster shot to help increase immunity.

Microbiologists and research-based physicians will also seek more information about how VZV works in the body and how the body responds to the virus.

While great strides have been made in discovering the basics of the disease, much more information is left to be discovered. Knowing, for example, the connection between age and shingles outbreak can help to predict who might and why he or she might get an outbreak of shingles. This might result in additional vaccine policy changes as needed to protect the public from shingles.

Epidemiologists will likely study the rates of the different strains of VZV that are causing disease in young people. For example, the Merck varicella vaccine uses a specifically grown variant in its vaccine, which is called the Oka/Merck strain. It has been shown to cause chicken pox and shingles in individuals who are exposed to those who have recently been vaccinated. It also has been documented to cause chicken pox in individuals who are recently vaccinated. Targeted research will be able to identify the specific strain to determine if the vaccine itself is causing an increase in chicken pox cases. Because scientists feel that artificially acquired immunity to VZV is safer than and just as effective as naturally acquired, they will be studying the rates of complication and death associated with each strain.

Scientists also need to establish better guidelines for both prevention and treatment for shingles and its complications. While the vaccine is available for almost all individuals (except those in special risk groups and those under 50 years old), its rates of success are only around 50%. Studies to determine the protection the immune system provides in naturally acquired and artificially acquired VZV could help to predict how best to prevent shingles from happening. This would be particularly beneficial for those individuals who need it most: the immune-compromised, pregnant, and those with cancer.

As the years progress and those who have had the varicella vaccination begin to reach the age where shingles might present, epidemiologists will need to derive a treatment specifically for them. Since the vaccine became commonplace in 1996, there have only been approximately 16 years worth of data related to widespread use of the vaccine. Once these individuals reach 50 years of age, their risk of developing shingles is unknown. Scientists are not sure how the immune system's response differs between natural and artificial immunity or how shingles will present when it reactivates in those with artificial immunity. Some data suggests that artificially immune adults will be at a lower risk for shingles, but there is no peer-reviewed data to confirm that. The amount of immunity conferred by the varicella vaccine is not yet known in widespread practice, but in the next 20 years, the results will be worth a clear, research-based study.

As the children who were vaccinated grow into maturity, the scientific community will be watching closely to see how the artificially immune hold up against the possibility of shingles. The dormant virus in their bodies is fundamentally different than a natural variety, and this may affect the outcome of its reactivation. Hopefully, with the administration of regular booster shots, much like tetanus, VZV infection will remain low and relatively safe to have.

Scientists might also develop a specific tool for identifying VZV in an office setting. Currently, the procedure for identifying shingles requires a blood draw and a complicated test to determine the causative agent. A delay of 14 days can make a big difference to those with shingles disease. With a simple rapid test, doctors could quickly identify the reason for the rash and not lose precious time before treating the individual. If antivirals are taken within 72 hours of the first sign of outbreak, the duration of the outbreak is considerably less than if the medicine is taken after 72 hours.

Scientists will also be studying the long-term safety of the shingles vaccine. While the clinical trials do suggest safety, the true test is widespread, long-term use of a product to determine actual risk. The Vaccine Adverse Event Reporting Service (VAERS) in conjunction with the CDC have established studies to look at the safety of the shingles vaccine as reported through the VAERS system.

Regardless of the choices that will be made by doctors and scientists in the future for shingles, patients must become aware of the choices available to them for all aspects of the disease. Treatments, vaccines and options for care will likely be thrust into the mainstream as more and more individuals surface with shingles every year.

Conclusion

Varicella zoster virus can sometimes seem secretive and elusive. Ruthlessly sought out by your immune system for years on end, it hides in the one place it knows the killer cells can't reach—the nervous system. Acting like a fugitive for many years, sometimes it overcomes the natural barriers in place to erupt in an ugly flower of pain that lasts for weeks, and in some cases years. It's difficult to come to terms with the concept that the virus that causes a mild case of chicken pox can later mete out its revenge on the skin of the unfortunate, but that is precisely what shingles disease does.

Shingles disease is caused by the varicella zoster virus as it reactivates from deep within the nervous tissue. As it migrates down the nerves, it brings with it pain, burning and itching. For many people living with shingles, the prospect of a life without shingles seems a distant memory. But, with appropriate treatment and attention, shingles disease need not be a life-threatening or dangerous condition. It is, however, an extremely painful condition that sometimes warrants close monitoring by a physician. Other times, shingles is completely manageable with just some aspirin. It's an unpredictable disease and one that many people take for granted.

Because of the often unrelenting discomfort, living with shingles can be painful and depressing. Individuals who have shingles should seek out the treatment they deserve and see that their pain is managed as best it can be. When one has shingles disease, it is not the time to be a hero and endure the burning pain for weeks. Shingles disease can be treated with antivirals, tricyclic antidepressants and analgesics or a combination of all three medications. Many people find that shingles becomes better with every day that passes until the reactivation has run its course.

While there is no cure for shingles, there is hope through education, scientific advancement and quality treatments that can reduce pain. Education about what shingles disease is, how to treat it and how to live with it can provide valuable information that might transform your shingles experience from traumatic to bearable.

www.ingramcontent.com/pod-product-compliance
Lightning Source LLC
Chambersburg PA
CBHW060001300526
45794CB00003B/1033